How to Overcome Eating Disorder

Recover from Eating Disorder and Control Emotional Eating
(Anorexia Nervosa, Bulimia, And Binge Eating)

By

Erika Robinson

Copyright © Erika Robinson – All rights reserved.

No part of this publication shall be reproduced, duplicated or transmitted in any way or by any means, digital or otherwise, including photocopying, scanning, uploading, recording and translating or by any information storage or retrieval system, without the written consent of the author.

"This book is not intended as a substitute for the medical advice of physicians. The reader should regularly consult a physician in matters relating to his/her health and particularly concerning any symptoms that may require diagnosis or medical attention."

Table of Contents

What is an Eating Disorder? 5

Types of Eating Disorders 8

What are the Causes of Eating Disorders? 14

Treatment Setting and their Types 24

Alternative Treatments for Eating Disorders 27

Anorexia Nervosa Eating Disorder 31

Bulimia Nervosa Eating Disorder 39

Binge Eating Disorder 49

Conclusion 57

What is an Eating Disorder?

The term eating disorder is used to describe an illness that is characterized by abnormal eating behavior and habits. These behaviors, in turn, cause severe changes and distress to the shape and weight of the body. A lot of people have misunderstood eating disorder to be an illness related to foods and lifestyle choices completely.

The fact: Eating disturbance and abnormalities are just symptoms of the condition. That means, it is not necessarily what the individual eat that leads to the illness; it is rather the other way around. For example, in cases of anorexia nervosa, it is a result of the inadequate food intake, that the individual's health and wellbeing gradually deteriorate.

According to research, eating disorders can be manifested in any individual - regardless of their age or gender. It occurs often in young adults and adolescents, but older adults and children are not left out.

Studies have observed common eating disorders among kids of 5 years and above. Eating disorders also manifest in adults of over 50 years, which means people of all age groupes are susceptible to eating disorder, with kids having the hihgest percentage.

Also, its symptoms are more experienced in women than men; and can manifest differently in each sex. For some men, it could be more of muscle size gain than weight loss.

More than just disrupting your daily activities, this illness can affect your emotional and mental health. For instance, there could be times you find yourself feeling unduly anxious about your calorie intake or embarrassed about your weight. This may cause you to isolate from people, just for expressing their concerns about your health. The incident may generally lead to depression as a further symptom.

Generally, the more the illness is allowed to linger and not addressed, the more significant the damage caused, like affecting your digestion, the skin, bones, reducing teeth and gum strength, and even the heart performance.

Types of Eating Disorders

Starting from anorexia, bulimia, to binge eating, all eating disorders should be treated with inherent attention. Ignoring some minor eating distortions can lead to chronic diseases, rooting from this eating disorders.

Anorexia Nervosa – when someone is obsessed about gaining weight and the fear of gaining weight and settles for self-starvation, the condition is referred to as anorexia nervosa.

This is not just a psychological condition, but potentially life-threatening. Most of the times, this obsession is usually unrealistic and untrue. So, in reality, they are underweight but feel they are overweight. Their perception of their weight is much more than what it is.

People with such disorder typically possess an extremely low body weight compared to their body type and height. This ultimately leads to a refusal in maintaining a balanced and proper consumption of food.

As a result of their fear of gaining weight, their bodies gradually get distorted. This illness is not really about consumption of food. It's a result of people's perception of themselves and an unhealthy way of coping with their emotions.

Symptoms usually related to this type of eating disorder are:

- Unhealthy weight gain
- Fear of weight gain
- False perception of body image and shape
- Undue efforts towards controlling weight
- Menstruation problems among females

Bulimia Nervosa - The Bulimia Nervosa sterns from a Greek word that means "ravenous hunger." It is an eating disorder that results from repeated binge eating or overeating and then afterward compensating with behaviors such as extreme and excessive exercise, forced vomiting, prolonged fasting, extreme diuretics, and laxatives.

All of these behaviors manifest to avoid weight gain and be in control. Individuals who have Bulimia are exposed to the effects of electrolytic imbalance such as severe dehydration, heart, and gastrointestinal problems.

Fluctuations of the body's weight also characterize this eating disorder. While the body's weight fluctuations (at an average 2-4 lbs. daily) are a common occurrence within individuals that are healthy, people with bulimia experience an abnormal fluctuation as a result of this chronic dieting.

Negative body image and low self-esteem tend to be on the top lists of the root causes of bulimia nervosa.

Even when they are afraid of weight gain, they still indulge in overeating - most of the times done secretly.

Symptoms associated with Bulimia are as follows:

- Cases of purging after binging
- Feeling of lack of control over your overeating
- Undue starving that eventually results in binging and purging
- Giving too much attention to your weight
- Embarrassed feeling concerning binging and purging
- Being secretive about your purging incidents

Binge Eating Disorder

This is a similar eating disorder to Bulimia - with frequent loss of control over eating, but unlike Bulimia, there is no compensatory behavior afterward. From time to time everyone overeats, and so detecting this illness is somewhat complicated. However, when it becomes too often and frequent, not necessarily for hunger, it is a sign that it's not normal.

As a result, a lot of binge eating disorder patients end up obese. They are also at high risk of developing conditions that have to do with the cardio. Most of the times, binge eating disorder is usually accompanied or preceded by feelings of shame; also, intense feelings of emotions such as distress, embarrassment, and guilt. If not properly addressed, it further influences the progress of the condition. Binge eating by itself is not necessarily bad but becomes a disorder when the individual loses control over eating.

Other than emotions, there are kinds of foods you consume that help in triggering binge episodes. This is true of carbohydrates. Foods high in fats and carbohydrates, according to scientists can trigger the release of the serotonin hormone in the brain, which in turn induces pleasurable emotions and feelings. And binge eaters always tend to gravitate towards such.

Symptoms of this eating disorder include:

- A tendency to overeat because of loss of control
- Feelings of shame and guilt after overeating
- Binge eating without any compensatory behavior
- Consuming more food than intended
- Secretive about overeating

What are the Causes of Eating Disorders?

Eating disorders are chronic illnesses that occur irrespective of age, gender, sex, race, and ethnicity. The good news is that they can be well treated. The problem with handling eating disorder is that the cause is not exactly known. However, there are a lot of contributing factors to the onset of the disease, and that still makes it complicated. Fortunately, certain causes have been established, some of which are psychological, biological and sociocultural. Below are listed some of these causes.

Biological Causes

Scientists have provided strong evidence that linked eating disorders to genetics. Some people possess genes that make them vulnerable to eating disorders. This genetic influence has been discovered to be a function of certain interactions between various genes, and not necessarily a particular gene. For this reason, the biological causes of eating disorder that relate to the gene are still not well understood.

Generally, having a parent or sibling who has once suffered from this condition increases your chances of also suffering from the disorder. Apart from genetics, there are co-morbidities related to mental health that accompany eating disorders, such as anxiety, depression, drug abuse, and the likes. These must be addressed so that they don't cause a recurrence.

Psychological Causes

Recent discoveries have concluded that personality traits also play a big role in the development of certain eating disorders. These theory angles towards anorexia and bulimia, being associated to modern influences.

These traits may be identified before the disorder incidence, during and after recovery.

These traits sum up the pieces of information psychologists consider determining the psychological treatment of a patient with an eating disorder. This usually has a way of complicating the decision-making process for the practitioners.

While each type of disorder has specific traits it associates with, there are also traits that apply to all. It is important to mention here that there are changes (such as behavior, interpersonal and cognition characteristics) that can be induced by prolonged starvation. This sometimes makes it very difficult to distinguish the cause from the effects.

Socio-cultural Causes

One of the common contributing factors leading to eating disorders is a sociocultural influence. Perceptions are easily gotten from the mass media such as magazine, television and other forms of advertising, as an ideal for beauty. These modern norms are usually false and misleading, especially to those with low self-esteem and lack of human support.

For instance, most cultures today project images that suggest and equate beauty with thinness and masculinity; with muscular and lean bodies - for females and males respectively. As these unrealistic ideals are internalized, people are more likely to develop dissatisfaction with their body, so it can lead to behaviors related to eating disorders. So, the more of these false perceptions are internalized, the higher the tendencies for an individual to fall into the hands of the eating disorder.

Personality Traits

There are a good number of personality traits, particularly during childhood that is connected to the development of eating disorders. As the child grows to adolescence, these traits become more strengthened due to influences like hormonal changes encountered during puberty and related stress and developments.

Traits such as emotional stability (also known as neuroticism), perfectionism and obsessiveness have been discovered to play a significant role in facilitating some eating disorders, especially bulimia and anorexia.

According to research, these traits are not necessarily driven by genetics. People with personality features that make them predisposed to emotions like anxiety, depression, perfectionism and self-criticism often encounter difficulty in eating healthy and managing a healthy weight. All of these increases the chances of triggering eating disorders.

Celiac Disease

One set of people that are more at risk of being affected by eating disorder illnesses are people with gastrointestinal disorders. It has been scientifically proven that there is a connection between anorexia nervosa with celiac disease. This implies that when a diagnosis of gastrointestinal is not properly attended to, it can alter their eating patterns - creating a food aversion (However, it is a complex process).

Related diseases such as inflammatory bowel disease and irritable bowel disease can also lead to developing the illness. This is particularly true of those overly conscious of their dietary intake. This has a way of making them consume foods that end up triggering the illness.

So, it is important that people with eating disorder be thoroughly evaluated for the presence of celiac, to avoid recurrence. Remember, the symptoms to look out for are the presence of gastrointestinal symptoms such as abdominal pain, diarrhea, distension, vomiting, decreased appetite, bloating.

Treatments for Eating Disorders

Although alternative medicine has developed popularity in the past decade, people still experience the effects of medications such as antidepressants and anti-anxiety medicines, among the combinations to tackle the phycological causes of eating distortions.

Medications are administered according to the severity and nature of the symptoms.

Generally, the goal(s) of an eating disorder treatment should be to address as much as possible, every aspect of the illness and restore the person to a healthy weight, and psychological and mental balance. Below are a few treatments and therapy that can help handle eating disorders.

Medication

Some medications are very helpful in handling an eating disorder. These medications are aimed at curbing urges or lessening thoughts about food that become obsessive. They help to reduce the urge to binge food, and the compensatory behavior that usually results after.

Medications have proven to be a viable intervention as they minimize or eradicate the possible mental conditions responsible for the underlying eating disorder. These medications include anti-anxiety agents or antidepressants.

In severe cases, this might not be enough to cure, but at least assists with the symptoms and stress component that promotes the disorder. As a general note, medications should generally not be the primary or initial treatment, particularly for anorexia nervosa type of the disorder. No specific medication has yet been approved, especially by the FDA for treating anorexia nervosa. So typically, the primary goal or objective, when medication is prescribed, is to help improve your weight.

Nutrition Prescription

We can agree that at the center of this illness is food and one's relationship with it. Therefore, it makes sense to say that nutrition therapy is a way forward toward a cure. Fondly referred to as Medical Nutrition Therapy (MNT), this method of treatment is holistic, as it aims at bringing to an end the various medical conditions and symptoms associated with emotional eating. To achieve this, registered dieticians put together a customized meal plan(s) that will help patients with their relationship with food and promote healthy eating behaviors.

Psychotherapy

Otherwise known as counseling or talk therapy, psychotherapy is an effective option for examining the behaviors and thoughts that are not just linked to the disorder but lead to it. The effectiveness of this method stairs from the fact that it allows the patients to be actively involved in the treatment. In the process, they don't just heal from traumatic life events, but learn vital skills for healthier coping and expressing of emotions, and thus maintaining healthy relationships.

This treatment includes cognitive behavioral therapy, where irrational thoughts about your self-image and body are examined and corrected where necessary. Family therapy also comes to play to when there is a need to improve family dynamics, reduce the stress that encourages eating disorders.

Treatment Setting and their Types

We have already established that treatment methods for eating disorders are approached according to the type and severity of the disorder. Depending on the stage of the illness and intensiveness of the condition, there are ways of receiving treatments.

Inpatient program

This is designed for serious cases of eating disorder, where the patient is already manifesting very serious symptoms that require thorough attention. Clinics that specialize on inpatient treatments are usually 24-hour care providers. The primary aim of this treatment is achieving medical stabilization, proper nourishment, and recovery of weight.

Outpatient Program

This is a program that is well-suited for people with mild symptoms of eating disorders. Even though they will still require specialized treatment from a health professional, they will not require intensive care and monitoring. For outpatients, there is usually an involvement from a group of health practitioners, and not necessarily one person staying in the hospital.

Day Program

This treatment program allows for more flexibility. This program is usually recommended when the severity of the illness is not worth worrying about. It involves different treatment sessions spread over the entire day or a certain number of days in a week. These sessions are flexible enough to hold in the comfort of the patient's home - as the case may be.

The programs and scheduling of the session are programmed in such a way the patient feels safe and supported.

Community-based Support

In recent times, community-based support groups have been emerging to help deal with medical conditions such as eating disorder and other associated conditions.

There are a good number of these support programs operating in local areas and providing information and support for people struggling with eating disorders. These organizations have been very helpful in handling a variety of issues relating to the eating disorder, its early intervention, and prevention.

Alternative Treatments for Eating Disorders

There has always been a debate as to how effective alternative therapy works. It is believed that traditional treatment for eating disorder as mentioned above are the most effective. However, times are fast changing, and alternative medicines and therapy are gradually becoming popular for various treatments. Since eating disorders are classified medically as psychological disorders that trigger negative effects, alternative therapy becomes an ideal approach, as it centers on the mind-body connection.

Acupuncture

This is one therapy that has in recent times gained traction in the treatment of eating disorders. Although the mechanisms behind the therapy are not fully understood, its usefulness cannot be denied. It is believed that if the insertion of the needles on strategic points in the body, through the skin, is properly done, a certain flow of life force and energy is balanced and improved, thereby eliminating various contributing factors to eating disorders.

Take, for instance, a hormone known as Leptin that helps in regulating the body's metabolism, and in reproductive function, together with a woman's menses.

Low level of the hormone leptin in women leads to period inhibition, which proves dangerous to health in the long-term. The first step to take, in this case, is to utilize methods of boosting the production of the leptin hormone such as acupuncture.

The discoveries are terrific and very promising in terms of dealing with the treatment of such disorder, and even other psychological distorting symptoms with similar root-cause. It has also been proven to be effective for treating conditions associated with eating disorders, such as depression and generalized anxiety.

Aromatherapy

Aromatherapy is basically the practice or the use of essential oils for healing. Essential oils are used to heal skin conditions, as well as mental conditions. Like any other alternative therapy, this treatment targets the underlying root cause of eating disorders. This treatment requires massaging the skin with oils or ingesting and inhaling them. The potential of this therapy is gradually being appreciated as more research is revealing more benefits of their methods. According to a certified aromatherapist, these essential oils are aimed at changing the emotional connection between people struggling with eating disorders and food. They do as much as address digestive and anxiety problems.

Naturopathy

One thing that is common among people with eating disorders, particularly anorexia or bulimia, is a deficiency of vitamins and minerals. One effective way to replenish the deficiencies, apart from nutrition prescription, is naturopathic therapy. This therapy comes in the form of supplements and herbs with the necessary ingredients handling the root cause of eating disorders.

To avoid unfavorable interaction of herbs and other drugs, you should consult your doctor before taking any herb, unless if you are not on any medication at the moment.

Anorexia Nervosa Eating Disorder

Generally speaking, all eating disorders are characterized by abnormal eating behaviors and an excessive drive for thinness, however, anorexia nervosa, as an eating disorder is a self-starvation syndrome that involves significant loss of weight - usually about 15 percent. With these, its treatment usually revolves around nutritional rehabilitation and behavioral monitoring; all aimed at normalizing body weight. Some of these treatments include:

Herbs

Herbs are a great way of strengthening and toning the body's systems. This therapy, like any other, should be done according to proper diagnosis and under the supervision of your doctor. These herbs can be used as dried extracts such as teas, powders or capsules, tinctures or glycerites. Also, these extracts can be taken alone or combined as will be directed by your doctor.

The tea extracts (1 teaspoon herb) are usually taken with a cup of hot water after steep-covered for about 10 minutes. Recommended intake is usually 2-4 cups every day. For tinctures, you have extracts such as Ashwagandha (for stress and general health benefits), Fenugreek (for appetite stimulation), Milk thistle (for liver health), catnip (soothing the digestive systems and calming the nerves).

You should exercise extreme caution when taking the extracts described. Certain medication should be avoided when you have cardiac conditions; as well as herbs, you may need to keep in contact with your doctor.

For example, people with tendencies for gastrointestinal ulcers are to avoid Ashwagandha, as they may irritate the gastrointestinal tract. You should not give Fenugreek to kids below 15 years.

It is not appropriate for those who have diabetes, as they may cause certain unhealthy interactions with other drugs in the system.

Dietary Supplements

People with anorexia nervosa usually tend towards being deficient in certain minerals and vitamins. The deficiencies of such minerals that serve as dietary supplements, can cause a detrimental effect to your system, physical, and mental health respectively.

According to studies, deficiencies in vitamins have a way of contributing to difficulties in cognitive abilities such as loss of memory and poor judgment. In other words, a great way of correcting these problems is ensuring an adequate intake of minerals and vitamins via diet or supplements.

Also, there are certain nutritional tips to take note of, such as:

- Avoid substances like alcohol, tobacco, and caffeine.

- Take at least seven glasses of bottled water every day, or any clean water.
- Ensure your protein are gotten from quality sources, such as eggs, meat, vegetable protein shakes, and wheat.
- Always avoid refined sugars or taking foods that contain high sugar content.

Suggested supplements for addressing nutritional deficiencies associated with anorexia nervosa include:

- A daily dose of multivitamin, particularly those containing the antioxidant vitamins like A, C, E, B-vitamins, and trace minerals, like calcium, magnesium, copper, selenium, phosphorus, and zinc.
- Also, a daily dose (usually 1 tsp or 2 capsules of omega-3 fatty acids like fish oil as it helps in improving immunity and decreasing inflammation. Other

good sources include cold water fishes like halibut or salmon.
- Coenzyme Q10 (100 to 200 mg) to be taken at bedtime, as it helps with muscular support, immunity and antioxidant properties.

Other supplements include a three times dosage (50 mg) of 5-hydroxytryptophan (5-HTP) for mood stabilization, a daily intake of creatine for muscle strengthening, probiotic supplement for immune and selectively, gastrointestinal health.

Acupuncture

One treatment that proven to be very effective in treating eating disorders, particularly the basic three of them, is the Chinese traditional medicine known as acupuncture. This treatment carries within it the ability to help regain physical and emotional health. According to health experts, eating disorders comes with certain medical complications associated with cardiac and endocrine systems. Furthermore, it impacts on the digestive system; and in fact, this is the most affected. This can be seen from systems of eating disorders such as abdominal bloating, acid reflux, diarrhea, constipation, irritable bowel syndrome and so on.

Here is how acupuncture helps in such related conditions:

Acupuncture as a treatment for eating disorder helps in addressing general health complaints such as fatigue, dry skin, anemia, concentration difficulties, muscle cramps, insomnia, low energy, and anxiety. So, when this therapy is employed, it initiates a speedy recovery of the systems of the body that have been affected.

Different and specific parts of the body are targeted, based on observed symptoms and determined treatment strategies, that will provide the most effective outcome. For instance, ear (auricular) acupuncture points are effective when it comes to harmonizing absorption, digestion, and metabolism.

Also, acupuncture body points (particularly the stomach) help in modifying or increasing the Chi energy, blood and oxygen circulation. In restoring the balance of the Chi energy, uncontrollable cravings and appetite can be managed by acupuncture.

Seek help

The recovery period for this illness is variable, usually fully recovered between 4 to 6 years. A high chance of relapse has also been observed after recovery. This is largely because patients keep it to themselves until it gets complicated. Because of the complicated state, only about 50% of anorexia nervosa patients recover from the illness; 25% never completely recover; unfortunately, about 20% lose their lives as a result of the complications of the condition. Sometimes, even after they have been termed "cured" still find themselves struggling. The high lifetime mortality rate associated with illness is alarming.

Bulimia Nervosa Eating Disorder

While anorexia deals with people with the tendency and likelihood to skip meals, adopt unhealthy and highly restrictive diets, bulimia deals with overeating or binging, followed by compensating with the use of laxatives and diuretics to purge and vomit. Like any other type of eating disorder, there are alternative treatments to medicines that can be used to help with bulimia nervosa.

Supplements

Like any illness, people suffering from bulimia nervosa eating disorder are most likely to fall short of certain minerals and nutrients. It is still not agreed that supplements completely get rid of bulimia, but one thing that is certain is these supplements help to improve the symptoms or conditions usually associated with the illness. These supplements are believed to contain the essential vitamins and minerals that the body needs to recover from the illness and complications that come with it.

Vitamins to look out for include:

Vitamin A: Otherwise known as beta carotene, are found in vegetables, liver and fish, yellow and green vegetables, and fruits; apricots, beets, butter, cheese, carrots, milk products, broccoli, cantaloupe, garlic, fresh mustard, red peppers, green olives, parsley, papaya, sweet potatoes, spinach, pumpkin, watercress, and asparagus. This vitamin has impacts on your appetite and the immune system of the body. Other parts such as eyes, bones, skin, soft tissues, teeth, and hair.

Vitamin B Complex: This vitamin is usually sourced from dairy products, nuts, meat, vegetables, nuts high in protein, brown rice, broccoli, cabbage, beans, cauliflower, eggs, cheese, fish, milk, poultry, meat, poultry, raisins, oatmeal, spinach, whole grains, peanut, yogurt and sprouts. This vitamin has impacts on your gastrointestinal tracts, liver, nervous system, and so on.

Vitamin B12: This is yet another essential vitamin and it's found in milk products, beef, cheese, fish, clams, mackerel, crab, kidney, eggs, liver, herring, seafood, and pork.

Massage

One effective component of any treatment of bulimia nervosa eating disorder is a therapeutic massage. According to studies carried out in the New York State University, people who included massage therapy as part of their treatment experience rapid and effective recovery from the illness. Massage helps to reduce depression, stress levels and anxiety in people suffering from eating disorders, and as such reduces dissatisfaction of the body and undue drive for perfectionism. The result is an improved self-image.

This therapy is known to boost the production of hormones such as serotonin and dopamine, thereby lowering stress levels and leaving the patients feeling calm and happier after the session. Massage is one therapy that seemed to be addressing the root of the problem with an eating disorder, which is their perception of themselves. Generally, this therapy fulfills the connection, according to psychologists, between self-esteem, body image, healthy social skills, with the need to be caressed and touched.

Herbs

Herbs are generally used to help people with eating disorders. However, there are specific herbs that are effective for bulimia nervosa patients.

With the use of these herbs, you regain strength, and you will have a happy gut. Your system will work properly and your craving for food, or junk food will be regulated.

It is important that a health care provider be informed about your condition and recommend possible treatment.

Holy basil: Otherwise known as Ocimum sanctum, is a standardized extract that helps to reduce stress. They can also be prepared in the form of teas. These herbs help in strengthening the effect of some blood thinners such as aspirin, Plavix (clopidogrel), and Coumadin (warfarin). It is also known to interact with sedatives such as pentobarbital (Nembutal).

Catnip: Otherwise known as Nepeta spp., is a tea that is aimed at calming the nerves of the digestive system and soothing them as well. This is also not recommended for pregnant and breastfeeding women, or those with the disease of the pelvis, except by doctors' approval.

Nutrition education

A lack of control over the amount of choice of food you eat is also an important symptom of bulimia nervosa.

People with this illness usually lose touch when it comes to their body's natural cues for hunger and fullness. This lack of proper inuitive decision-making affects personal food intake regulation. So, food habits are basically distorted upon such disability.

Therefore, regaining that sense of control is central to boosting self-efficacy and confidence and thereby overcoming urges to recurrently binge and compensate with purging. Also, taking in a nutritionally rich and balanced diet is very important for the recovery of a bulimic patient.

Any holistic treatment program should include nutrition education and meal planning, as one of its components. This is aimed at repairing the damage done to the body by unhealthy eating habits and also developing healthy ones.

Foods recommended for bulimia nervosa include whole grains, such as popcorn, brown rice, barley, wild rice, bulgur, rye, and bulgur. Another includes probiotics gotten from sources such as yogurt, buttermilk, sour cream, fermented miso kefir, and sauerkraut.

Also essential are omega-3 fatty acids sourced from fatty fish such as tuna, salmon, sardines and mackerel, as well as canola oil, ground flax seeds, walnut oil, and flaxseed oil. All of these is to help in adequately nourishing your body and then possibly reversing signs of malnourishment resulting from bulimia eating disorder.

Acupuncture

Some experts are of the opinion that acupuncture is not a promising treatment, but the majority believe that the effect of this treatment has the potential of being topmost on the list. It has existed for centuries in Traditional Chinese Medicine, and every day there's been an improvement in the therapy.

Even though there is no solid scientific proof behind the working of this therapy for treating bulimia, the results that have been so far registered can speak for it. Acupuncture has also been very instrumental in the treatment of addictive behaviors.

To increase the chances of success with the therapy, it must be done by a highly trained acupuncturist, who recommends the treatment based on an individual's unique condition. Generally, including acupuncture, the treatment plan for bulimia increase the recovery speed and performance of the treatment.

Ask for help

Often, people who have bulimia are ashamed to disclose their condition and as such tend to manage the condition unaddressed for many years. As this continues to happen, their habits gradually get harder to change. The more complicated the situation gets, the more difficult and time-consuming it is to treat.

It is very important that the moment you begin to observe abnormal eating behaviors or symptoms of eating disorder like bulimia, you should talk to your doctor. The doctor will now get you examined and checked for physical signs of the conditions, such as a salivary enlarging, trace of depression and thin tooth enamel.

Another area that will be looked into is the person's weight, mental and physical health and exercise habits. With early diagnosis and treatment, relapse after treatment and mortality incidence is minimized.

Binge Eating Disorder

People often confuse binge eating with bulimia because of their similarities. However one thing that differentiate them is that binge eating does not involve compensating with a purge after excessively consuming food. One useful help with this illness is natural treatments. They play a great role in overcoming the disorder. Since binge eating and bulimia manifest similarly, the treatment naturally involves similar therapies.

Nutrition

Nutrition is an important element of any treatment plan for binge eating disorder, as it helps to address the body's health - physically, behavioral and emotional. Nutrition here is aimed at normalizing the eating behaviors by providing nutrients and calories in their sufficient amounts.

An appropriate diet for compulsive overeating aims to provide nutrients that will help regulate binge cravings. This diet is to supply healthy foods from all food group and meet the requirements of a basic healthy diet. Even foods from lean protein, complex carbohydrate sources and healthy type of fats.

Don't hesitate to include raw vegetables and high-quality protein as this helps to prolong times of eating and improved satiation respectively. Appropriate amounts of food should be dished and slowly eaten, and in an atmosphere that is pleasurable for eating and enhancing control over portion consumed.

It is important to ensure ample consumption of water to stay adequately hydrated. Remember, all of these helps to keep food cravings at bay, to avoid triggering episodes of binge eating. Some of the foods to go for are whole grains such as oatmeal, wild rice, air-popped corn, and brown rice, in the place of foods like pasta, cereals, snack foods and bread.

For protein sources, go for legumes, egg whites, fish and fat-low diary product in place of processed and fatty red meat. Sources of healthy fat include olive oil, nuts, canola oil, seeds, avocados, and salmon.

Supplements

It is true that the exact cause(s) of binge eating disorder are yet to be known. However clues suggest that it is associated with psychological distress. Minerals and multivitamins as supplements play a role in enhancing the body's chemicals. This helps in controlling the urge to eat in excess.

Magnesium Glycinate (500 mg): This helps in calming the brain, and the body as a way to ensure stabilization of the glucose level usually fluctuated after binge eating.

According to a recent research, "stability of magnesium and food cravings are closely related, in essence."

L-Glutamine (500 mg): Usually taken three times daily, this amino acid helps to control wild sugar cravings. Usually comes in the form of a capsule, it converts to brain food when taken.

Prebiotics: Yes, prebiotics, and not probiotics. Prebiotics help to reduce depression and anxiety. They impact on bacteria housed in your gut and tampering the chemistry of your brain.

5-HTP (200 mg): This is one supplement when taken subdues any urge to binge. It helps to suppress any form of appetite and then makes you relaxed, thereby eliminating any anxiety and tendency to binge.

Trace Minerals

There are numerous trace minerals and are important for enhancing brain function and human health, but there are three of the essentials and particularly directed at disturbance that root from binge eating disorder. Briefly, they are chromium, for regulating glucose and controlling depression symptoms; magnesium, for fighting hunger, anxiety and depression; and zinc, to help eliminate depression and restore your appetite to normal.

Zinc

The mineral known as zinc plays an essential role in the development and growth of the body, as well as its neurological function, reproduction, neurotransmitter synthesis, and immune response.

Various important enzymic reactions are dependent on the availability of zinc in the body. Its other essential functions include DNA synthesis, production of proteins, cell division, wound healing and bone growth.

It is important that this mineral be consumed every day since the human body is unable to store it. One of the symptoms of its deficiency is depression.

Chromium

When chromium levels in the body are inadequate, the result is an increase in carbohydrate cravings, depression, hypoglycemia, and impaired glucose tolerance. This mineral is an essential component of glucose tolerance factor, a dietary agent that enhances the ability of insulin to move blood sugar into cells.

Simply put, chromium works together with receptors of insulin featured on the cells and creates room for the entrance of glucose. This means that when this mineral is absent in the body, it affects the effectiveness of insulin and how the body handles glucose. This, in turn, results in a high craving for carbohydrate or sugar and increased in hunger.

Magnesium

The role of magnesium is so vital, as it features in a lot of metabolic processes in the body, this includes the conversion of fat, carbohydrates (into energy). Also, this mineral is required for the function of over 300 enzymes, such as those responsible for neurotransmitters synthesis - for instance, serotonin. Symptoms common with lack of magnesium include insomnia, headaches, fatigue, constipation, sugar cravings, insulin resistance, and premenstrual syndrome.

Ask for help

Binge eating is probably the most common eating disorder and very dangerous too. As much as possible you want to avoid it. However, if you see yourself struggling with the condition, one thing you must consider is that you're not alone, and there is a way out of it. Sometimes fighting your way through it without help can be futile, you want to get help from a certified and qualified health professional.

Do not fall into the trap most people do and be ashamed of opening up and seeking help. The earlier the condition is diagnosed and treated, the easier and faster it is to treat. The good news remains that a good number of people successfully recover from binge eating without much struggle.

Conclusion

Eating disorder is generally life-threatening, particularly with Anorexia Nervosa and Bulimia Nervosa.

Through the combination of medical treatments and therapy, one can get to manage and treat the symptoms that come with the illness. Unfortunately, a lot of people with eating disorders fail to receive treatment. There are men and women with these disorders appearing as though they are just struggling in life.

Sometimes or most times, people with this illness are not aware of it. They think it's a normal experience until it gets worse. Also, because of the secrecy associated with this illness, particularly the bulimia, it usually goes unnoticed even by family members and friends.

Early diagnosis is an advantage for a quick recovery. The moment any symptoms associated with this illness is noticed, make every possible effort to see your physician. Your physician is expected to ask you a couple of questions that have to do with your eating and exercising and purging habits. And also, how frequent it has been.

In consulting with a physician, you should provide every detail and try to be honest with your feelings and disease history. It is very important for a professional to understand the underlying causes, so he would have more leverage for tackling the illness.

Early treatment also significantly reduces any chances of complications.

Books by the Same Author

1. Cognitive Behavioral Therapy Techniques: How to Manage Anxiety and Depression Using CBT – Control Your Thinking, Emotions, and Behavior

2. Intermittent Fasting for Women: How to Lose Weight Without Exercise, Boost Energy, Reverse Diabetes, And Prevent Cancer – Slow Down the Aging Process

3. Ketogenic Diet for Beginners: Simple Keto Recipes and Diet Plan to Lose Fat, Heal Your Body, and Boost Energy

4. Adrenal Fatigue Solution: Powerful Methods to Boost Your Energy, Improve Metabolism, And Stimulate Your Hormones

5. How to Reverse Fibromyalgia Cookbook: Recipes and Meal Plan to Relieve Symptoms and Treat Root Cause

6. How to Reverse Hashimoto's Thyroiditis: Eliminate Root Cause and Heal Hypothyroidism Symptoms Naturally

7. CBD Hemp Oil Beginners Guide: The Healing Benefits of Cannabidiol Essential Oil

8. Paleo Diet Cookbook: Nutritional Recipes to Boost Health and Prevent Toxicity

www.ingramcontent.com/pod-product-compliance
Lightning Source LLC
LaVergne TN
LVHW040044040226
830973LV00010B/573